GYNECOLOGY
101
Medical Key Terms and Interesting Tidbits

Damian O.

Cook

Copyright

Contents

INTRODUCTION

Gynecology is a branch of medicine dedicated to women's health, specifically focusing on the reproductive system. It plays an essential role in helping women understand their bodies, manage their health, and navigate life changes from puberty through menopause and beyond. Gynecologists not only address concerns related to menstruation, fertility, and pregnancy but also treat a range of conditions like ovarian cysts, endometriosis, and polycystic ovary syndrome (PCOS), which can impact daily life if left untreated.

An appointment with a gynecologist often involves a general health check, as well as specific exams to screen for diseases like cervical cancer. One common procedure is the Pap smear, a test that checks for abnormal cells in the cervix, potentially detecting early signs of cancer. In recent years, more advanced screening methods, like HPV testing, have become standard alongside Pap smears, improving the chances of catching issues early.

But gynecology is not just about addressing problems; it's also about education. Many gynecologists spend time answering questions about sexual health, contraception, and family planning, empowering women to make informed decisions. This open communication helps to dispel myths and encourage women to take control of their health confidently.

The field of gynecology has advanced significantly in recent decades. Today, minimally invasive surgeries, like laparoscopy, have become popular for treating certain conditions, allowing for quicker recovery times and less pain. This is a far cry from the treatments available in the past, reflecting how gynecology has embraced technology to improve patient care.

Overall, gynecology is a vital field that supports women's health and well-being across their lives. By normalizing regular check-ups and encouraging open dialogue about health concerns, gynecologists help women lead healthier, more empowered lives. Listed below is the compilation of some of the key terms used in the gynecology field.

The Key Terms

Abruption Placentae

Abruption placentae is a medical emergency where the placenta detaches from the uterine wall before birth, depriving the fetus of oxygen and nutrients.

------ **Interesting FACT**: Abruption placentae can lead to severe maternal bleeding and fetal distress, often requiring an emergency cesarean section to save the baby and mother.

Adenocarcinoma of the Endometrium

Adenocarcinoma of the endometrium is the most common type of uterine cancer, developing in the lining of the uterus and often linked to excess estrogen exposure.

------ **Interesting FACT**: Early-stage adenocarcinoma of the endometrium has a high survival rate if detected and treated promptly, usually with surgery.

Adenomyosis

Adenomyosis is a condition where the inner lining of the uterus breaks through the muscle wall of the uterus, leading to heavy periods and pelvic pain.

------ **Interesting FACT**: Adenomyosis typically resolves after menopause and is more common in women who have had children.

Alpha-Fetoprotein (AFP)

Alpha-fetoprotein is a protein produced by the fetal liver, and high levels of AFP in the mother's blood can indicate neural tube defects or other developmental issues in the fetus.

------ **Interesting FACT**: AFP is measured during the second trimester as part of prenatal screening, and abnormal levels may prompt further testing like amniocentesis.

Amenorrhea

Amenorrhea is the absence of menstruation during a woman's reproductive years. It can be classified as primary (when menstruation never begins) or secondary (when periods stop after having occurred previously).

------ **Interesting FACT**: Female athletes, especially those in endurance sports like long-distance running or gymnastics, are more prone to developing amenorrhea due to intense physical training and reduced body fat.

Amniocentesis

Amniocentesis is a procedure in which a small amount of amniotic fluid is withdrawn from the uterus for testing, often used to detect genetic abnormalities in the fetus.

------ **Interesting FACT**: Amniocentesis is usually performed between the 15th and 20th weeks of pregnancy and carries a slight risk of miscarriage.

Androgen Insensitivity Syndrome (AIS)

Androgen insensitivity syndrome is a genetic condition where a person who is genetically male (XY chromosomes) is resistant to male hormones (androgens), leading to the development of female physical traits despite having male chromosomes.

------ **Interesting FACT**: Individuals with AIS are usually raised as girls and may not realize they have the condition until puberty when menstruation does not occur.

Anembryonic Pregnancy

Anembryonic pregnancy, also known as a blighted ovum, occurs when a fertilized egg implants in the uterus but fails to develop into an embryo.

------ **Interesting FACT**: Anembryonic pregnancy is a leading cause of early pregnancy loss and is often detected through an ultrasound showing an empty gestational sac.

Anovulation

Anovulation is the absence of ovulation, meaning an egg is not released from the ovary during the menstrual cycle, leading to irregular periods and potential infertility.

------ **Interesting FACT**: Anovulation is common in conditions like polycystic ovary syndrome (PCOS) and can often be treated with medications to induce ovulation, such as clomiphene citrate.

Aromatase Inhibitors

Aromatase inhibitors are drugs used to lower estrogen levels in postmenopausal women by blocking the enzyme aromatase, which converts androgens into estrogen, often used in breast cancer treatment.

------ **Interesting FACT**: Aromatase inhibitors are commonly prescribed for hormone-receptor-positive breast cancer, especially in postmenopausal women, as estrogen can fuel the growth of some breast cancers.

Asherman's Syndrome

Asherman's syndrome is a condition characterized by scar tissue or adhesions forming inside the uterus, often as a result of surgery like a D&C, leading to reduced menstrual flow or infertility.

------ **Interesting FACT**: Asherman's syndrome is a leading cause of secondary infertility and may require surgical treatment to remove the adhesions.

Atrophic Vaginitis

Atrophic vaginitis is the thinning and inflammation of the vaginal walls due to a decrease in estrogen, most often occurring after menopause, causing symptoms like dryness and irritation.

------ **Interesting FACT**: Hormonal treatments like estrogen creams or vaginal moisturizers are often used to alleviate the discomfort associated with atrophic vaginitis.

Bacterial Vaginosis (BV)

Bacterial vaginosis is a common vaginal infection caused by an imbalance of naturally occurring bacteria, leading to symptoms like a thin, gray discharge and a fishy odor. ------ **Interesting FACT**: BV is not a sexually transmitted infection, but it is more common in sexually active women, and treatment typically involves antibiotics.

Bartholin's Cyst

A Bartholin's cyst is a fluid-filled swelling of the Bartholin's glands, which are located on either side of the vaginal opening and help lubricate the vagina. ------ **Interesting FACT**: If a Bartholin's cyst becomes infected, it can develop into an abscess, requiring drainage or surgical removal to alleviate pain and discomfort.

Bicornuate Uterus

A bicornuate uterus is a congenital uterine abnormality

where the uterus is heart-shaped with two separate cavities, increasing the risk of miscarriage and preterm labor.

------ **Interesting FACT**: Many women with a bicornuate uterus can carry a pregnancy to term, though surgical correction may be required in some cases to improve pregnancy outcomes.

Cervical Cerclage

Cervical cerclage is a surgical procedure in which the cervix is stitched closed during pregnancy to prevent premature birth or miscarriage.

------ **Interesting FACT**: Cervical cerclage is typically performed for women with a weak or incompetent cervix and is usually done between 12 and 14 weeks of pregnancy.

Cervical Dysplasia

Cervical dysplasia refers to abnormal changes in the cells of the cervix, which can be detected through a Pap smear and may lead to cervical cancer if left untreated.

------ **Interesting FACT**: Cervical dysplasia is often caused by human papillomavirus (HPV) infection, and regular Pap smears can help detect it early before it progresses to cancer.

Cervical Incompetence

Cervical incompetence refers to a cervix that dilates prematurely during pregnancy, often leading to miscarriage or preterm birth.

------ **Interesting FACT**: Cervical incompetence is often treated with a cervical cerclage, a procedure in which the cervix is stitched closed to prevent early dilation.

Cervical Polyp

A cervical polyp is a small, benign growth on the cervix, often causing light bleeding or spotting, particularly after intercourse or between periods.

------ **Interesting FACT**: Cervical polyps are common in

women over the age of 40 and are usually noncancerous, but they are often removed to ensure they are benign.

Cervicitis

Cervicitis is the inflammation of the cervix, often caused by infections such as chlamydia or gonorrhea, and can lead to symptoms like vaginal discharge, pain, or bleeding.

------ **Interesting FACT**: Cervicitis is commonly treated with antibiotics, and if left untreated, it can lead to pelvic inflammatory disease (PID) and infertility.

Chlamydia

Chlamydia is a common sexually transmitted infection caused by the bacterium *Chlamydia trachomatis*, often asymptomatic but capable of causing serious reproductive health issues if left untreated.

------ **Interesting FACT**: Chlamydia is easily treated with antibiotics, but if left untreated, it can lead to pelvic

inflammatory disease (PID) and increase the risk of
infertility.

Chorioamnionitis

Chorioamnionitis is an infection of the fetal membranes
(chorion and amnion) during pregnancy, often caused by
bacteria entering the uterus, leading to fever and uterine
tenderness.

------ **Interesting FACT**: Chorioamnionitis is a major cause
of preterm birth and can lead to complications for both
the mother and baby if untreated.

Choriocarcinoma

Choriocarcinoma is a rare but aggressive type of cancer
that develops from the cells of the placenta, often after a
molar pregnancy, miscarriage, or childbirth.

------ **Interesting FACT**: Choriocarcinoma is highly
treatable with chemotherapy, especially when detected
early, and it can spread to other organs, such as the lungs
or brain.

Chorionic Gonadotropin

Chorionic gonadotropin is a hormone produced by the placenta during pregnancy that helps maintain the corpus luteum, which in turn supports early pregnancy by producing progesterone.

------ **Interesting FACT**: Human chorionic gonadotropin (hCG) is the hormone detected in home pregnancy tests, and its levels increase rapidly in early pregnancy.

Chorionic Villus Sampling (CVS)

Chorionic villus sampling is a prenatal test where a sample of placental tissue is taken to detect chromosomal abnormalities in the fetus.

------ **Interesting FACT**: CVS can be performed earlier than amniocentesis, usually between the 10th and 13th weeks of pregnancy, providing earlier genetic information.

Chronic Pelvic Pain

Chronic pelvic pain is persistent pain in the pelvic region

lasting for six months or more, often caused by conditions like endometriosis or interstitial cystitis.

------ **Interesting FACT**: Chronic pelvic pain affects millions of women worldwide, and it can be difficult to diagnose due to its association with various gynecological and gastrointestinal conditions.

Clomiphene Citrate

Clomiphene citrate is a medication used to stimulate ovulation in women with infertility due to ovulatory disorders, such as polycystic ovary syndrome (PCOS).

------ **Interesting FACT**: Clomiphene citrate is often used as a first-line treatment for infertility and has been successful in helping many women conceive by promoting the release of eggs from the ovaries.

Colporrhaphy

Colporrhaphy is a surgical procedure to repair a defect in the vaginal wall, often performed to treat pelvic organ prolapse.

------ **Interesting FACT**: Colporrhaphy can be performed to fix either a cystocele (bladder prolapse) or rectocele (rectal prolapse) and helps restore normal vaginal anatomy.

Colposcopy

Colposcopy is a procedure used to closely examine the cervix, vagina, and vulva for signs of disease, often after abnormal Pap smear results.

------ **Interesting FACT**: Colposcopy allows for real-time viewing of potentially precancerous cells and can involve taking biopsies for further analysis.

Corpus Luteum Cyst

A corpus luteum cyst forms after an egg is released from the ovary and the corpus luteum (the structure left behind) fills with fluid, sometimes causing pelvic pain or delaying the start of the next menstrual period.

------ **Interesting FACT**: Most corpus luteum cysts resolve on their own without treatment, but in rare cases, they can cause complications such as ovarian torsion or rupture.

Cystadenoma

Cystadenoma is a benign tumor that develops in the ovaries, filled with fluid or mucus, and can grow quite large, causing discomfort or pressure in the abdomen.
------ **Interesting FACT**: Cystadenomas can weigh several pounds and may require surgical removal, but they are noncancerous and typically don't spread.

Cystocele

A cystocele occurs when the bladder drops into the vagina due to weakened pelvic floor muscles, leading to symptoms like urinary incontinence or a feeling of pressure in the pelvic area.
------ **Interesting FACT**: Cystocele is common in women who have had multiple vaginal deliveries, and treatments range from pelvic floor exercises to surgery, depending on the severity.

Decidual Cast

A decidual cast occurs when the entire lining of the uterus sheds in one large piece, often causing cramping and heavy bleeding.

------ **Interesting FACT**: Decidual casts are relatively rare and can be mistaken for a miscarriage, although they are not directly related to pregnancy loss.

Dermoid Cyst

A dermoid cyst is a benign ovarian tumor that contains various types of tissues, such as hair, skin, and teeth, because it arises from germ cells.

------ **Interesting FACT**: Dermoid cysts are also called mature cystic teratomas and can grow quite large, although they are typically noncancerous.

Dilation and Curettage (D&C)

Dilation and curettage is a procedure in which the cervix is dilated, and the lining of the uterus is scraped or suctioned out for diagnostic or therapeutic purposes.

------ **Interesting FACT**: D&C is often performed after a miscarriage or to diagnose conditions like uterine polyps or abnormal bleeding.

Dysfunctional Uterine Bleeding (DUB)

Dysfunctional uterine bleeding refers to abnormal bleeding from the uterus that is not related to menstruation, pregnancy, or any recognizable pelvic disease.

------ **Interesting FACT**: DUB is often caused by hormonal imbalances and is most common during adolescence and perimenopause.

Dysmenorrhea

Dysmenorrhea is the medical term for painful menstrual cramps that occur before or during a period.

------ **Interesting FACT**: Dysmenorrhea is one of the most common gynecological complaints, affecting more than half of menstruating women.

Dyspareunia

Dyspareunia refers to pain during sexual intercourse, which can be caused by physical or psychological factors, including infections, vaginal dryness, or anxiety.

------ **Interesting FACT**: Dyspareunia is more common in postmenopausal women due to hormonal changes leading to vaginal dryness, but it can affect women of any age.

Eclampsia

Eclampsia is a serious complication of pregnancy that involves seizures in a woman with preeclampsia (high blood pressure and organ damage), which can be life-threatening for both the mother and baby.

------ **Interesting FACT**: Eclampsia is considered a medical emergency and usually requires immediate delivery of the baby to prevent further complications.

Ectopic Pregnancy

An ectopic pregnancy occurs when a fertilized egg implants outside the uterus, usually in a fallopian tube, and can be life-threatening if not treated.

------ **Interesting FACT**: Ectopic pregnancies account for about 1-2% of all pregnancies and cannot result in a live birth.

Endocervical Curettage

Endocervical curettage is a procedure where tissue is scraped from the endocervical canal to test for abnormal or cancerous cells, often following an abnormal Pap smear.

------ **Interesting FACT**: This procedure is often used to detect cervical dysplasia or early-stage cervical cancer and is performed during a colposcopy.

Endocervical Polyp

An endocervical polyp is a benign growth in the cervical

canal, which may cause irregular bleeding or discharge, especially in postmenopausal women.

------ **Interesting FACT**: These polyps are generally harmless, but doctors usually remove them to prevent symptoms or potential complications.

Endocervicitis

Endocervicitis is the inflammation of the inner lining of the cervix, often caused by bacterial infections like chlamydia or gonorrhea, leading to vaginal discharge or bleeding.

------ **Interesting FACT**: Untreated endocervicitis can lead to more severe conditions like pelvic inflammatory disease (PID), which may result in infertility.

Endometrial Ablation

Endometrial ablation is a procedure to remove or destroy the lining of the uterus (endometrium) to reduce heavy menstrual bleeding.

------ **Interesting FACT**: Endometrial ablation is considered a minimally invasive alternative to hysterectomy, but it is not suitable for women who wish to become pregnant in the future.

Endometrial Cancer

Endometrial cancer is a type of cancer that begins in the lining of the uterus (endometrium), often presenting with abnormal vaginal bleeding, especially after menopause. ------ **Interesting FACT**: Endometrial cancer is the most common type of uterine cancer, and early detection through abnormal bleeding increases the chances of successful treatment.

Endometrial Hyperplasia

Endometrial hyperplasia is the thickening of the endometrial lining, often caused by excess estrogen without progesterone. ------ **Interesting FACT**: If left untreated, endometrial hyperplasia can increase the risk of developing endometrial cancer.

Endometrial Polyp

An endometrial polyp is a growth in the lining of the uterus, often causing abnormal uterine bleeding or infertility.

------ **Interesting FACT**: Endometrial polyps are usually benign, but about 1% of them may develop into cancer, which is why they are often removed and analyzed.

Endometrioma

An endometrioma is a type of cyst formed when endometrial tissue grows in the ovaries, often associated with endometriosis and causing pelvic pain.

------ **Interesting FACT**: Endometriomas are sometimes called "chocolate cysts" because they are filled with old, dark blood.

Endometriosis

Endometriosis occurs when tissue similar to the lining of the uterus (endometrium) grows outside the uterus, causing pain, heavy periods, and potential fertility issues.

------ **Interesting FACT**: Endometriosis can affect the ovaries, fallopian tubes, and pelvic lining, and while there is no cure, treatments include pain relief and hormonal therapies.

Endosalpingitis

Endosalpingitis is the inflammation of the inner lining of the fallopian tubes, often caused by bacterial infections, and can lead to infertility if untreated.

------ **Interesting FACT**: Endosalpingitis is often associated with pelvic inflammatory disease (PID) and may result from sexually transmitted infections such as chlamydia or gonorrhea.

Epidural Anesthesia

Epidural anesthesia is a common form of pain relief used during labor, administered through a catheter placed in the lower back to numb the lower half of the body.

------ **Interesting FACT**: While epidurals are highly effective at reducing labor pain, they can sometimes slow down labor or cause temporary drops in blood pressure.

Episiotomy

An episiotomy is a surgical cut made at the opening of the vagina during childbirth to help the baby pass through more easily, preventing severe tearing.

------ **Interesting FACT**: Episiotomies were once routine during childbirth but are now less common, as research has shown that natural tears may heal better.

Fallopian Tubes

The fallopian tubes are the pair of tubes that carry eggs from the ovaries to the uterus, and fertilization typically occurs within these tubes.

------ **Interesting FACT**: Blocked fallopian tubes are a common cause of infertility, and conditions like ectopic pregnancies occur when the fertilized egg implants in the tube instead of the uterus.

Fetal Distress

Fetal distress refers to signs that a fetus is not well, often due to oxygen deprivation, and it may lead to an emergency delivery to prevent harm to the baby.

------ **Interesting FACT**: Fetal distress is often detected through abnormal fetal heart rate patterns during labor, and immediate intervention, such as a cesarean section, may be required.

Fibroadenoma

A fibroadenoma is a benign breast tumor that is made up of both glandular and fibrous tissue, commonly found in women under the age of 30.

------ **Interesting FACT**: Fibroadenomas are usually painless and can feel like a firm, smooth lump in the breast, but they do not increase the risk of breast cancer.

Fibrocystic Breast Disease

Fibrocystic breast disease is a benign condition in which a

woman's breasts feel lumpy or rope-like due to fibrous tissue and cyst formation, often associated with hormonal changes.

------ **Interesting FACT**: Fibrocystic breast changes are common and typically worsen just before menstruation, but they are not associated with an increased risk of breast cancer.

Fibroid

A fibroid is a noncancerous growth that develops in or around the uterus, often causing heavy menstrual bleeding or discomfort.

------ **Interesting FACT**: Fibroids are more common in African-American women, who tend to develop them at younger ages and experience more severe symptoms.

Fistula

A fistula is an abnormal connection between two body parts, such as between the vagina and rectum, which can occur after childbirth or surgery.

------ **Interesting FACT**: Obstetric fistulas are most common in areas with limited access to obstetric care, often resulting from prolonged labor, and can be surgically repaired.

Follicle-Stimulating Hormone (FSH)

Follicle-stimulating hormone is produced by the pituitary gland and plays a crucial role in regulating the menstrual cycle and stimulating the growth of ovarian follicles.

------ **Interesting FACT**: FSH levels are measured in fertility tests to assess a woman's ovarian reserve and ability to conceive, particularly during fertility treatments.

Follicular Cyst

A follicular cyst is a benign cyst that forms on an ovary when a follicle fails to release an egg and continues to grow, usually resolving on its own.

------ **Interesting FACT**: Follicular cysts are common and usually harmless, though larger cysts may cause pelvic pain or pressure and require medical attention.

Galactorrhea

Galactorrhea is the spontaneous flow of milk from the breast, unrelated to childbirth or breastfeeding, and is often caused by excessive prolactin production.

------ **Interesting FACT**: Galactorrhea can occur in both men and women and is often a sign of a pituitary tumor (prolactinoma) or side effect of certain medications.

Gestational Diabetes

Gestational diabetes is a type of diabetes that develops during pregnancy, characterized by high blood sugar levels that can affect both the mother and baby.

------ **Interesting FACT**: Women who develop gestational diabetes have a higher risk of developing type 2 diabetes later in life, and their babies are at increased risk for obesity and glucose intolerance.

Gonadotropins

Gonadotropins are hormones that stimulate the ovaries,

often used in fertility treatments to promote ovulation.

------ **Interesting FACT**: The two main gonadotropins are follicle-stimulating hormone (FSH) and luteinizing hormone (LH), both critical for regulating the menstrual cycle.

Gonorrhea

Gonorrhea is a sexually transmitted infection (STI) caused by the bacterium *Neisseria gonorrhoeae*, which can infect the reproductive tract, causing symptoms like pain and discharge.

------ **Interesting FACT**: If untreated, gonorrhea can lead to pelvic inflammatory disease (PID) in women, increasing the risk of infertility and ectopic pregnancy.

Granulosa Cell Tumor

A granulosa cell tumor is a rare type of ovarian tumor that arises from granulosa cells, which are involved in the production of sex hormones like estrogen.

------ **Interesting FACT**: Granulosa cell tumors can cause early puberty in girls or abnormal uterine bleeding in women due to excess estrogen production.

Hematocolpos

Hematocolpos is the accumulation of menstrual blood in the vagina, often caused by an obstruction, such as an imperforate hymen.

------ **Interesting FACT**: Hematocolpos can lead to pelvic pain and abdominal swelling, and treatment typically involves surgery to remove the blockage and allow menstrual flow.

Hematometra

Hematometra is the accumulation of blood in the uterus, often caused by a blockage in the cervix, which can result in severe pelvic pain.

------ **Interesting FACT**: Hematometra may occur after certain gynecological procedures or due to congenital abnormalities, and it is usually treated by surgically removing the obstruction.

Hematosalpinx

Hematosalpinx is the presence of blood in a fallopian tube, often caused by a ruptured ectopic pregnancy or pelvic inflammatory disease (PID).

------ **Interesting FACT**: Hematosalpinx is a medical emergency if caused by an ectopic pregnancy and requires immediate surgical intervention to prevent serious complications.

Hemorrhagic Cyst

A hemorrhagic cyst is a type of ovarian cyst that occurs when a blood vessel in the wall of the cyst breaks, causing blood to fill the cyst.

------ **Interesting FACT**: Hemorrhagic cysts are usually benign and may cause pelvic pain, particularly if they rupture, but they often resolve on their own.

Herpes Simplex Virus (HSV)

Herpes simplex virus is a common sexually transmitted

infection that causes sores, typically around the mouth (HSV-1) or genitals (HSV-2).

------ **Interesting FACT**: Once infected with HSV, the virus remains in the body and can reactivate, causing recurrent outbreaks of sores.

Human Chorionic Gonadotropin (hCG)

Human chorionic gonadotropin is a hormone produced during pregnancy by the placenta, and it helps maintain the corpus luteum to support the early stages of pregnancy.

------ **Interesting FACT**: hCG is the hormone detected by home pregnancy tests, and its levels are also monitored in certain fertility treatments and conditions like molar pregnancies.

Human Papillomavirus (HPV)

HPV is a common sexually transmitted infection that can cause genital warts and is the leading cause of cervical cancer.

------ **Interesting FACT**: There are over 100 types of HPV, and the virus can affect both men and women, but vaccines are available to prevent the most dangerous strains.

Hydatidiform Mole

A hydatidiform mole is a type of gestational trophoblastic disease in which a nonviable pregnancy forms abnormal tissue growths, resembling a bunch of grapes, instead of a fetus.

------ **Interesting FACT**: Hydatidiform mole is part of a group of conditions known as molar pregnancies and can lead to a rare form of cancer called choriocarcinoma if not treated.

Hydrosalpinx

Hydrosalpinx refers to a fallopian tube that is blocked and filled with fluid, often caused by infection or inflammation, which can lead to infertility.

------ **Interesting FACT**: Hydrosalpinx is commonly treated with surgery to remove the affected tube or with procedures to drain the fluid and restore fertility.

Hymenectomy

Hymenectomy is the surgical removal of the hymen, typically performed if the hymen is abnormally thick or causing discomfort.

------ **Interesting FACT**: Hymenectomy is sometimes performed in cases of an imperforate hymen, where the hymen completely blocks the vaginal opening, preventing menstruation.

Hyperemesis Gravidarum

Hyperemesis gravidarum is a severe form of morning sickness, characterized by excessive nausea and vomiting during pregnancy, leading to dehydration and weight loss.

------ **Interesting FACT**: Hyperemesis gravidarum affects about 1-2% of pregnant women and can require hospitalization for IV fluids and nutritional support.

Hypermenorrhea

Hypermenorrhea refers to abnormally heavy or prolonged menstrual bleeding, often caused by conditions like fibroids, hormonal imbalances, or clotting disorders.

------ **Interesting FACT**: Hypermenorrhea can lead to anemia if left untreated and is often managed with medications, hormonal therapy, or surgery depending on the underlying cause.

Hypomenorrhea

Hypomenorrhea refers to unusually light menstrual bleeding, which can result from hormonal imbalances, birth control use, or structural abnormalities in the uterus.

------ **Interesting FACT**: Hypomenorrhea can be a sign of polycystic ovary syndrome (PCOS) or thyroid disorders, but it can also occur naturally during perimenopause.

Hysterectomy

A hysterectomy is the surgical removal of the uterus, sometimes including the cervix, ovaries, and fallopian tubes, and it may be performed for a variety of medical reasons, such as fibroids, cancer, or endometriosis.

------ **Interesting FACT**: Hysterectomy is one of the most common surgeries for women, and while it eliminates the risk of uterine cancer, it also permanently ends menstruation and the ability to become pregnant.

Hysterosalpingectomy

Hysterosalpingectomy is the surgical removal of the uterus and fallopian tubes, typically performed to treat uterine cancer or other severe gynecological conditions.

------ **Interesting FACT**: This procedure is more extensive than a hysterectomy alone and may be performed if there is concern about the spread of cancer to the fallopian tubes.

Hysterosalpingogram (HSG)

A hysterosalpingogram is an X-ray procedure used to examine the uterus and fallopian tubes, often performed to check for blockages that could cause infertility.

------ **Interesting FACT**: HSG involves injecting a contrast dye into the uterus and fallopian tubes, which helps identify structural problems or blockages that may interfere with conception.

Hysteroscopy

Hysteroscopy is a procedure that uses a thin, lighted tube inserted through the vagina and cervix to examine the inside of the uterus, often used to diagnose and treat abnormal bleeding.

------ **Interesting FACT**: Hysteroscopy can also be used to remove fibroids or polyps, and is considered a minimally invasive alternative to more extensive surgeries.

Imperforate Hymen

An imperforate hymen is a congenital condition where the hymen completely covers the vaginal opening, preventing the passage of menstrual blood and other fluids.

------ **Interesting FACT**: An imperforate hymen is typically diagnosed at puberty when a girl does not have periods despite the development of other secondary sexual characteristics, and it is corrected with surgery.

Incompetent Cervix

An incompetent cervix is a condition in which the cervix begins to open (dilate) too early during pregnancy, increasing the risk of miscarriage or preterm birth.

------ **Interesting FACT**: An incompetent cervix is often treated with a cerclage, a surgical procedure in which the cervix is stitched closed to help prevent preterm birth.

Interstitial Cystitis

Interstitial cystitis is a chronic bladder condition that causes pelvic pain, pressure, and urinary urgency, often mistaken for a urinary tract infection.

------ **Interesting FACT**: The cause of interstitial cystitis is unknown, and it primarily affects women, making it challenging to treat, with symptoms varying widely among patients.

Interstitial Pregnancy

An interstitial pregnancy is a type of ectopic pregnancy where the fertilized egg implants in the portion of the fallopian tube that passes through the uterine wall, a condition that can be life-threatening if ruptured.

------ **Interesting FACT**: Interstitial pregnancies are rare but more dangerous than other ectopic pregnancies due to the proximity to the uterus and potential for heavy bleeding.

Intrauterine Adhesions

Intrauterine adhesions, also known as Asherman's syndrome, occur when scar tissue forms inside the uterus, often after surgery, leading to reduced menstrual flow or infertility.

------ **Interesting FACT**: Intrauterine adhesions can be treated with hysteroscopic surgery to remove the scar tissue and improve fertility outcomes.

Intrauterine Device (IUD)

An intrauterine device (IUD) is a small, T-shaped device inserted into the uterus to prevent pregnancy, either through hormonal or copper mechanisms.

------ **Interesting FACT**: IUDs are one of the most effective forms of reversible contraception and can last for several years depending on the type.

Kallmann Syndrome

Kallmann syndrome is a genetic disorder that causes

delayed or absent puberty due to a lack of production of certain hormones needed for sexual development, often linked to a deficiency in gonadotropin-releasing hormone (GnRH).

------ **Interesting FACT**: Kallmann syndrome can also affect the sense of smell (anosmia), and fertility treatments are often required to induce puberty and reproductive function.

Labiaplasty

Labiaplasty is a surgical procedure to reshape or reduce the size of the labia, often done for cosmetic reasons or to relieve discomfort.

------ **Interesting FACT**: Labiaplasty has become one of the most popular cosmetic surgeries in recent years, but it can also be performed for medical reasons, such as to reduce irritation or pain.

Laparoscopy

Laparoscopy is a minimally invasive surgical procedure in

which a small camera (laparoscope) is inserted into the abdomen through a small incision to view the pelvic organs or perform surgical procedures.

------ **Interesting FACT**: Laparoscopy is commonly used to diagnose or treat conditions such as endometriosis, ovarian cysts, or ectopic pregnancy, and it allows for quicker recovery compared to open surgery.

Laparotomy

A laparotomy is a surgical procedure involving a large incision in the abdomen to examine the abdominal organs, often used to diagnose or treat gynecological conditions like ovarian cysts or fibroids.

------ **Interesting FACT**: Laparotomy is sometimes necessary when less invasive procedures like laparoscopy cannot provide enough access to the pelvic organs for treatment or diagnosis.

Leiomyoma

Leiomyoma, commonly known as fibroids, are benign

tumors that grow in the uterus' smooth muscle tissue.

------ **Interesting FACT**: While fibroids are non-cancerous, they are the leading cause of hysterectomies in women in the United States.

Leiomyosarcoma

Leiomyosarcoma is a rare and aggressive cancer of the smooth muscle cells, most commonly affecting the uterus.

------ **Interesting FACT**: Unlike uterine fibroids, which are benign, leiomyosarcomas are malignant and can spread to other parts of the body, requiring aggressive treatment.

Lichen Sclerosus

Lichen sclerosus is a skin condition affecting the vulva, causing white patches, itching, and discomfort, and can lead to scarring if untreated.

------ **Interesting FACT**: Lichen sclerosus is more common in postmenopausal women and can increase the risk of vulvar cancer.

Luteal Phase Defect

Luteal phase defect is a condition where the second half of the menstrual cycle (the luteal phase) is too short or has insufficient progesterone, affecting fertility.

------ **Interesting FACT**: Women with luteal phase defects may struggle to maintain a pregnancy due to the uterus not being properly prepared for embryo implantation.

Luteal Phase

The luteal phase is the second half of the menstrual cycle, occurring after ovulation and lasting until menstruation begins. During this time, the body prepares for potential pregnancy by increasing progesterone production.

------ **Interesting FACT**: A short luteal phase, known as luteal phase defect, can cause difficulty in maintaining a pregnancy due to inadequate progesterone levels.

Luteinizing Hormone (LH)

Luteinizing hormone is a hormone produced by the pituitary gland that triggers ovulation and the production of progesterone in the ovaries.

------ **Interesting FACT**: LH levels surge during the middle of the menstrual cycle, and this surge is what ovulation predictor kits detect to identify fertile days.

Mammoplasty

Mammoplasty refers to surgical procedures to change the size or shape of the breasts, including breast augmentation or reduction.

------ **Interesting FACT**: Mammoplasty is not only performed for cosmetic reasons but can also be used for reconstructive purposes, such as after a mastectomy.

Mastalgia

Mastalgia refers to pain in the breast, which can occur due to hormonal changes, injury, or infections.

------ **Interesting FACT**: Cyclical mastalgia, which is linked to the menstrual cycle, is the most common type of breast pain, often intensifying before menstruation.

Mayer-Rokitansky-Küster-Hauser Syndrome (MRKH)

MRKH is a rare congenital condition where the uterus and upper part of the vagina are underdeveloped or absent, while external genitalia and ovaries remain normal.

------ **Interesting FACT**: Women with MRKH typically have normal ovarian function and secondary sexual characteristics but cannot carry a pregnancy.

Menarche

Menarche refers to a girl's first menstrual period, marking the onset of puberty.

------ **Interesting FACT**: The average age of menarche has decreased over time due to factors such as improved nutrition and health care, now occurring around age 12 in many countries.

Menometrorrhagia

Menometrorrhagia is a condition characterized by abnormally heavy and prolonged menstrual bleeding that occurs at irregular intervals.

------ **Interesting FACT**: Menometrorrhagia can be caused by hormonal imbalances, uterine fibroids, or polyps, and may require treatment with medications or surgery.

Mittelschmerz

Mittelschmerz is a term used to describe the one-sided pelvic pain that occurs around the time of ovulation, often felt as a sharp or cramping sensation.

------ **Interesting FACT**: The word "mittelschmerz" is German for "middle pain," as the discomfort occurs in the middle of the menstrual cycle during ovulation.

Molar Pregnancy

A molar pregnancy is a rare complication of pregnancy where abnormal tissue grows in the uterus instead of a normal embryo. It can be a complete or partial molar pregnancy, depending on whether any normal fetal tissue is present.

------ **Interesting FACT**: Molar pregnancies can lead to a rare type of cancer called choriocarcinoma and require prompt removal of the abnormal tissue.

Mucinous Cystadenoma

Mucinous cystadenoma is a benign ovarian tumor that is filled with a thick, mucous-like fluid and can grow to a large size, sometimes causing abdominal discomfort.

------ **Interesting FACT**: Although benign, mucinous cystadenomas can become quite large and may require surgical removal to prevent complications such as ovarian torsion.

Mullerian Agenesis

Mullerian agenesis is a congenital condition where a woman is born without a fully developed uterus or vagina, which can cause infertility or lack of menstruation.

------ **Interesting FACT**: Women with Mullerian agenesis usually have normal external genitalia and ovaries, and the condition is often discovered when menstruation does not begin during puberty.

Myomectomy

A myomectomy is a surgical procedure to remove uterine fibroids (leiomyomas) while preserving the uterus, often performed to relieve symptoms like heavy bleeding or pelvic pain.

------ **Interesting FACT**: Unlike a hysterectomy, which removes the entire uterus, myomectomy allows women to retain their fertility, making it an option for women who want to have children.

Oligohydramnios

Oligohydramnios is a condition characterized by a deficiency of amniotic fluid surrounding the fetus during pregnancy, which can lead to complications such as growth restriction or preterm birth.

------ **Interesting FACT**: Oligohydramnios can be caused by fetal anomalies, placental insufficiency, or rupture of membranes, and may require close monitoring or early delivery.

Oligomenorrhea

Oligomenorrhea is infrequent or very light menstruation, typically occurring in cycles longer than 35 days.

------ **Interesting FACT**: Oligomenorrhea can result from conditions such as polycystic ovary syndrome (PCOS) or significant weight loss.

Oophorectomy

Oophorectomy is the surgical removal of one or both

ovaries.

------ **Interesting FACT**: An oophorectomy can reduce the risk of ovarian cancer, particularly for women with BRCA gene mutations.

Oophoritis

Oophoritis is the inflammation of one or both ovaries, often caused by infections, and can lead to pelvic pain and potential fertility issues.

------ **Interesting FACT**: Oophoritis is sometimes associated with pelvic inflammatory disease (PID) and can result from bacterial infections, such as tuberculosis or mumps.

Ovarian Cancer

Ovarian cancer is a malignant tumor that begins in the ovaries, and it is often not detected until it has spread to other areas, making it difficult to treat.

------ **Interesting FACT**: Ovarian cancer is sometimes called the "silent killer" because its symptoms, like bloating or pelvic pain, are often vague and easily overlooked in its early stages.

Ovarian Cyst

An ovarian cyst is a fluid-filled sac that forms on or inside an ovary, which can cause pain or discomfort but is often harmless.

------ **Interesting FACT**: Most ovarian cysts are functional, meaning they form as part of the normal menstrual cycle, and often disappear on their own.

Ovarian Hyperplasia

Ovarian hyperplasia is the abnormal enlargement of the ovarian cells, which can lead to an increased risk of developing ovarian cancer.

------ **Interesting FACT**: Ovarian hyperplasia is often associated with conditions like polycystic ovary syndrome (PCOS) and can cause hormonal imbalances.

Ovarian Hyperstimulation Syndrome (OHSS)

OHSS is a complication that can occur when the ovaries are overstimulated during fertility treatments, causing them to swell and leak fluid into the abdomen.

------ **Interesting FACT**: OHSS can range from mild to severe, and in extreme cases, it can cause dangerous complications like blood clots, kidney failure, or fluid buildup in the chest.

Ovarian Reserve

Ovarian reserve refers to a woman's remaining supply of eggs and is an important factor in fertility, as a lower reserve may reduce the chances of conception.

------ **Interesting FACT**: Ovarian reserve can be assessed through blood tests measuring anti-Müllerian hormone (AMH) levels and antral follicle counts via ultrasound.

Ovarian Torsion

Ovarian torsion occurs when an ovary twists around the

ligaments that hold it in place, cutting off its blood supply and causing severe pain and potentially damaging the ovary.

------ **Interesting FACT**: Ovarian torsion is a medical emergency and often requires immediate surgery to untwist or remove the affected ovary to prevent tissue damage.

Pelvic Exenteration

Pelvic exenteration is an extensive surgical procedure to remove the reproductive organs, bladder, and parts of the rectum to treat advanced pelvic cancers.

------ **Interesting FACT**: Pelvic exenteration is usually a last-resort surgery for cancer that has spread in the pelvic area, and it dramatically alters a patient's anatomy and quality of life.

Pelvic Girdle Pain (PGP)

Pelvic girdle pain is discomfort in the pelvic joints during pregnancy, affecting mobility and making everyday activities like walking or climbing stairs difficult.

------ **Interesting FACT**: About 20% of pregnant women experience pelvic girdle pain, and it can persist after childbirth in some cases, though physical therapy can help.

Pelvic Inflammatory Disease (PID)

Pelvic Inflammatory Disease is an infection of the female reproductive organs, often caused by sexually transmitted infections like chlamydia or gonorrhea.

------ **Interesting FACT**: PID can lead to long-term complications like infertility or chronic pelvic pain if not treated promptly.

Pelvic Organ Prolapse (POP)

Pelvic organ prolapse occurs when the muscles and tissues supporting the pelvic organs weaken, allowing the bladder, uterus, or rectum to drop into the vagina.

------ **Interesting FACT**: Pelvic organ prolapse is common in women who have had multiple vaginal deliveries and can cause urinary incontinence or discomfort, sometimes requiring surgery.

Pelvic Ultrasound

A pelvic ultrasound is an imaging test that uses sound waves to create pictures of the organs in the pelvic area, such as the uterus, ovaries, and fallopian tubes, to detect abnormalities.

------ **Interesting FACT**: Pelvic ultrasounds are often used to diagnose conditions like ovarian cysts, uterine fibroids, and early pregnancy complications.

Pelvimetry

Pelvimetry is the measurement of the dimensions of the pelvis, often used to assess whether a woman's pelvis is large enough for a vaginal birth.

------ **Interesting FACT**: While pelvimetry was once a common practice, it is now less frequently used due to advances in obstetric care, and most women can attempt vaginal birth regardless of pelvic size.

Perimenopausal Bleeding

Perimenopausal bleeding refers to irregular or heavy menstrual bleeding that occurs during the transition to menopause, often caused by fluctuating hormone levels.

------ **Interesting FACT**: Perimenopausal bleeding can sometimes mimic symptoms of other conditions like fibroids or endometrial hyperplasia, requiring further medical evaluation.

Perimenopause

Perimenopause is the transitional period leading up to menopause, during which hormone levels fluctuate, causing symptoms like irregular periods, hot flashes, and mood changes.

------ **Interesting FACT**: Perimenopause can last several years, and the average age of onset is in the mid-40s, though some women may experience it earlier or later.

Perineal Tear

A perineal tear is a tear in the perineum, the area between the vagina and anus, often occurring during childbirth. Tears are classified by degrees, with first-degree being the least severe and fourth-degree the most severe, extending to the anal canal.

------ **Interesting FACT**: Perineal tears are more common in women delivering their first baby, and a controlled delivery can help minimize the risk.

Perineorrhaphy

Perineorrhaphy is the surgical repair of the perineum, often performed after childbirth when the area has been torn or cut during delivery.

------ **Interesting FACT**: Episiotomy, a surgical cut made during delivery to widen the vaginal opening, may require perineorrhaphy for repair.

Peritoneal Carcinomatosis

Peritoneal carcinomatosis refers to the spread of cancer cells to the peritoneum, the lining of the abdominal cavity, often seen in advanced ovarian cancer.

------ **Interesting FACT**: Peritoneal carcinomatosis is usually diagnosed at an advanced stage, and treatment often involves surgery and chemotherapy to manage symptoms and slow progression.

Pessary

A pessary is a medical device inserted into the vagina to support pelvic organs, often used to treat pelvic organ prolapse or urinary incontinence.

------ **Interesting FACT**: Pessaries come in different shapes and sizes, and they are a non-surgical option for women with prolapse, allowing them to manage symptoms effectively.

Placenta Accreta

Placenta accreta occurs when the placenta attaches too deeply into the uterine wall, causing complications during delivery due to difficulties separating the placenta.

------ **Interesting FACT**: Placenta accreta is a life-threatening condition that can lead to severe hemorrhaging and often requires a cesarean section for delivery.

Placenta Previa

Placenta previa is a condition where the placenta covers part or all of the cervix, increasing the risk of severe bleeding during pregnancy and delivery.

------ **Interesting FACT**: Placenta previa is more common in women who have had multiple pregnancies or previous cesarean deliveries and often requires delivery by cesarean section.

Placental Abruption

Placental abruption is a serious condition in which the placenta detaches from the uterine wall before childbirth, depriving the baby of oxygen and nutrients.

------ **Interesting FACT**: Placental abruption occurs in about 1 in 100 pregnancies and can lead to preterm birth or stillbirth if not treated immediately.

Placental Insufficiency

Placental insufficiency occurs when the placenta cannot provide enough oxygen and nutrients to the fetus, leading to growth restrictions and potential pregnancy complications.

------ **Interesting FACT**: Placental insufficiency is a common cause of intrauterine growth restriction (IUGR) and may require early delivery to protect the health of the baby.

Polycystic Ovary Syndrome (PCOS)

PCOS is a hormonal disorder characterized by irregular menstrual periods, excess androgen levels, and the presence of multiple small cysts on the ovaries.

------ **Interesting FACT**: PCOS is one of the most common causes of infertility, affecting 6-12% of women of reproductive age, and can increase the risk of developing type 2 diabetes and cardiovascular disease.

Polycystic Ovary

A polycystic ovary contains multiple small, fluid-filled sacs or cysts, which can result from hormonal imbalances and is often associated with polycystic ovary syndrome (PCOS).

------ **Interesting FACT**: Polycystic ovaries can appear on imaging even in women without PCOS, making the syndrome a more complex diagnosis that includes symptoms like irregular periods and high androgen levels.

Polymenorrhea

Polymenorrhea refers to menstrual cycles that occur more frequently than every 21 days, leading to more frequent periods.

------ **Interesting FACT**: Polymenorrhea is often caused by hormonal imbalances, including thyroid disorders or perimenopause, and may require medical treatment to regulate the cycle.

Polypectomy

Polypectomy is the surgical removal of polyps, which are abnormal growths of tissue, often found in the uterus or cervix and can cause abnormal bleeding.

------ **Interesting FACT**: Polyps are usually benign but can sometimes develop into cancer, so they are often removed and examined for abnormalities.

Postmenopausal Bleeding

Postmenopausal bleeding refers to any vaginal bleeding that occurs after a woman has gone through menopause and can be a sign of conditions like endometrial cancer, polyps, or hormone imbalances.

------ **Interesting FACT**: Any postmenopausal bleeding should be evaluated by a doctor, as it can be an early sign of uterine or cervical cancer.

Pre-eclampsia

Pre-eclampsia is a serious pregnancy complication characterized by high blood pressure and signs of damage to organs, usually occurring after 20 weeks of pregnancy.

------ **Interesting FACT**: Pre-eclampsia affects 5-8% of pregnancies and, if untreated, can progress to eclampsia, which causes seizures and is potentially life-threatening for both the mother and baby.

Premature Ovarian Failure (POF)

Premature ovarian failure, also known as primary ovarian insufficiency, is a condition where the ovaries stop functioning before the age of 40, leading to early menopause.

------ **Interesting FACT**: POF affects approximately 1% of women under 40 and can result in infertility, though some women may still have occasional periods and even conceive.

Prolactinoma

A prolactinoma is a benign tumor of the pituitary gland that causes overproduction of prolactin, leading to symptoms such as irregular periods, milk production in non-pregnant women, and infertility.

------ **Interesting FACT**: Prolactinomas are the most common type of pituitary tumor and are typically treated with medication to reduce prolactin levels or, in some cases, surgery.

Pseudocyesis

Pseudocyesis, also known as a "false pregnancy," is a condition in which a woman believes she is pregnant, showing many of the physical symptoms, but there is no actual pregnancy.

------ **Interesting FACT**: Pseudocyesis is rare and can be linked to psychological factors, such as extreme desire or fear of pregnancy. Symptoms can include missed periods, morning sickness, and abdominal enlargement.

Puerperium

Puerperium refers to the period following childbirth, lasting about six weeks, during which the mother's body recovers and returns to a non-pregnant state.

------ **Interesting FACT**: During the puerperium, it is crucial for new mothers to monitor for signs of postpartum complications such as infections, hemorrhage, or depression.

Rectocele

Rectocele is a condition where the tissue between the rectum and vagina weakens, causing the rectum to bulge into the vaginal wall.

------ **Interesting FACT**: Rectocele often occurs in women who have had vaginal deliveries, particularly multiple or difficult births. May require surgical repair if symptoms are severe.

Rectovaginal Fistula

A rectovaginal fistula is an abnormal connection between the rectum and vagina, often resulting from childbirth, surgery, or disease, causing fecal matter to pass through the vagina.

------ **Interesting FACT**: Rectovaginal fistulas require surgical repair, and are more common in areas with limited access to healthcare, particularly after prolonged labor.

Retroverted Uterus

A retroverted uterus is a uterus that tilts backward instead of its usual forward position, which can cause discomfort or pain during intercourse or menstruation.

------ **Interesting FACT**: About 1 in 5 women have a retroverted uterus, and in most cases, it does not affect fertility or pregnancy outcomes.

Round Ligament Pain

Round ligament pain is a common pregnancy discomfort caused by the stretching of the round ligaments that support the uterus, often felt as sharp or jabbing pain in the lower abdomen or hip area.

------ **Interesting FACT**: Round ligament pain typically occurs in the second trimester and is caused by the rapid growth of the uterus, especially during movement.

Sacrocolpopexy

Sacrocolpopexy is a surgical procedure used to treat pelvic organ prolapse, where the vagina is lifted and attached to the sacrum to restore its normal position.

------ **Interesting FACT**: Sacrocolpopexy is often used to correct vaginal prolapse in women who have undergone a hysterectomy and is considered a highly effective treatment for pelvic organ prolapse.

Salpingectomy

Salpingectomy is the surgical removal of one or both fallopian tubes, often performed to treat ectopic pregnancies or reduce cancer risk.

------ **Interesting FACT**: Some women at high risk for ovarian cancer may choose to have a salpingectomy as a preventive measure.

Salpingitis Isthmica Nodosa (SIN)

Salpingitis isthmica nodosa is a condition where small nodules form in the fallopian tubes, leading to blockages and increased risk of ectopic pregnancy or infertility.

------ **Interesting FACT**: SIN is often diagnosed via hysterosalpingography (HSG) and can result in infertility if not treated, typically through surgery to open the blocked tubes.

Salpingitis

Salpingitis is the inflammation of a fallopian tube, often

caused by sexually transmitted infections like chlamydia or gonorrhea, and can lead to scarring and infertility.

------ **Interesting FACT**: Salpingitis is a significant cause of ectopic pregnancies because the damaged fallopian tube may prevent the fertilized egg from reaching the uterus.

Salpingostomy

Salpingostomy is a surgical procedure to create an opening in a blocked fallopian tube, often used to treat ectopic pregnancies or other fertility issues.

------ **Interesting FACT**: Salpingostomy can help preserve the fallopian tube in cases of ectopic pregnancy, unlike salpingectomy, which involves removing the tube entirely.

Sclerotherapy

Sclerotherapy is a procedure used to treat varicose veins or spider veins by injecting a solution that causes the veins to collapse and fade over time.

------ **Interesting FACT**: Sclerotherapy is often used as a cosmetic treatment to reduce the appearance of spider veins, especially in the legs, but it can also alleviate discomfort from larger varicose veins.

Septate Uterus

A septate uterus is a congenital abnormality where a fibrous or muscular septum divides the uterine cavity, which can increase the risk of miscarriage or preterm labor.

------ **Interesting FACT**: Women with a septate uterus often undergo surgery called hysteroscopic resection to remove the septum and improve pregnancy outcomes.

Sertoli-Leydig Cell Tumor

A Sertoli-Leydig cell tumor is a rare ovarian tumor that can produce male hormones, leading to symptoms like excessive hair growth or deepening of the voice in women.

------ **Interesting FACT**: Sertoli-Leydig cell tumors are usually benign but can become malignant in rare cases,

and they are often treated with surgery to remove the
tumor.

Sheehan's Syndrome

Sheehan's syndrome is a rare condition that occurs when
severe blood loss during childbirth damages the pituitary
gland, leading to hormone deficiencies and problems
such as infertility or difficulty breastfeeding.

------ **Interesting FACT**: Sheehan's syndrome can result in
lifelong hormonal replacement therapy if the pituitary
gland fails to recover its ability to produce hormones.

Skene's Glands

Skene's glands, also known as the paraurethral glands, are
located near the urethra and are believed to play a role in
female ejaculation.

------ **Interesting FACT**: Skene's glands are sometimes
referred to as the "female prostate" due to their
similarities in structure and function to the male prostate
gland.

Sonohysterography

Sonohysterography is an ultrasound procedure in which saline is injected into the uterus to better visualize the uterine cavity and detect abnormalities such as fibroids or polyps.

------ **Interesting FACT**: Sonohysterography provides clearer images than standard ultrasound and is often used when abnormal uterine bleeding is present or in cases of infertility.

Spontaneous Abortion

Spontaneous abortion, commonly known as miscarriage, is the loss of a pregnancy before the 20th week, often due to chromosomal abnormalities in the fetus.

------ **Interesting FACT**: Around 10-20% of known pregnancies end in spontaneous abortion, though many occur before a woman even knows she is pregnant.

Stein-Leventhal Syndrome

Stein-Leventhal syndrome is another term for polycystic ovary syndrome (PCOS), characterized by multiple ovarian cysts, irregular periods, and elevated androgen levels.

------ **Interesting FACT**: Stein-Leventhal syndrome was first described in 1935 by American gynecologists Irving Stein and Michael Leventhal and is now commonly referred to as PCOS.

Stillbirth

Stillbirth is the death of a fetus after 20 weeks of pregnancy but before delivery, resulting in the birth of a baby without signs of life.

------ **Interesting FACT**: Stillbirth affects about 1 in 160 pregnancies in the U.S., and risk factors include maternal conditions like diabetes, high blood pressure, and infections.

Struma Ovarii

Struma ovarii is a rare type of ovarian tumor made up of thyroid tissue, which can cause hyperthyroidism due to excess thyroid hormone production.

------ **Interesting FACT**: Although struma ovarii is an ovarian tumor, it can produce symptoms of hyperthyroidism, such as rapid heart rate, weight loss, and anxiety.

Submucosal Fibroid

A submucosal fibroid is a type of uterine fibroid that grows beneath the lining of the uterus, often causing heavy menstrual bleeding and potential fertility issues.

------ **Interesting FACT**: Submucosal fibroids can be removed surgically through a procedure called hysteroscopic myomectomy, which preserves the uterus and improves fertility.

Subserosal Fibroid

A subserosal fibroid is a type of uterine fibroid that grows on the outer wall of the uterus and may cause pressure on surrounding organs, leading to discomfort.

------ **Interesting FACT**: Subserosal fibroids are less likely to affect fertility compared to fibroids that grow inside the uterus but can still cause symptoms like bloating and pelvic pain.

Suction Curettage

Suction curettage is a procedure in which the contents of the uterus are removed using suction, commonly performed after a miscarriage or as an abortion method.

------ **Interesting FACT**: Suction curettage is one of the most common methods used to complete a miscarriage or for early elective abortions and can be done up to 12-14 weeks of pregnancy.

Teratocarcinoma

Teratocarcinoma is a malignant tumor that contains various types of tissues, such as muscle, hair, or bone, and can arise in the ovaries or testicles.

------ **Interesting FACT**: Teratocarcinomas are part of a group of tumors known as germ cell tumors, and they can be aggressive, often requiring surgery and chemotherapy.

Teratoma

A teratoma is a type of ovarian tumor that can contain different types of tissue, including hair, skin, and teeth, often benign but sometimes malignant.

------ **Interesting FACT**: Teratomas are sometimes referred to as "monster tumors" because they can contain a variety of tissue types, making them unusual in appearance.

Theca Lutein Cyst

A theca lutein cyst is a functional ovarian cyst that forms

due to overstimulation by elevated levels of human chorionic gonadotropin (hCG), often seen in molar pregnancies.

------ **Interesting FACT**: Theca lutein cysts are usually benign and resolve on their own after hCG levels decrease but can cause abdominal discomfort or pain.

Thecoma

Thecoma is a rare, benign ovarian tumor that originates from the theca cells of the ovary and often produces estrogen, which can lead to abnormal uterine bleeding.

------ **Interesting FACT**: Thecomas are most common in postmenopausal women and are usually treated with surgery to remove the tumor.

Toxic Shock Syndrome (TSS)

Toxic shock syndrome is a rare but life-threatening bacterial infection often associated with tampon use, causing high fever, rash, and organ failure.

------ **Interesting FACT**: TSS is caused by toxins produced by Staphylococcus aureus or Streptococcus bacteria and can also occur after surgery or skin infections.

Transabdominal Ultrasound

Transabdominal ultrasound is an imaging procedure where a probe is placed on the abdomen to visualize the pelvic organs, commonly used during pregnancy to monitor the fetus.

------ **Interesting FACT**: Transabdominal ultrasounds are often used in conjunction with transvaginal ultrasounds for clearer views of the uterus and ovaries, especially in early pregnancy.

Transvaginal Ultrasound

A transvaginal ultrasound is an imaging procedure where a probe is inserted into the vagina to get clearer images of the uterus, ovaries, and fallopian tubes.

------ **Interesting FACT**: Transvaginal ultrasounds are often used in early pregnancy to confirm the location of the pregnancy and detect fetal heartbeat, as well as to diagnose conditions like ovarian cysts or uterine fibroids.

Trichomoniasis

Trichomoniasis is a sexually transmitted infection caused by the parasite *Trichomonas vaginalis*, leading to symptoms such as itching, burning, and vaginal discharge. ------ **Interesting FACT**: Trichomoniasis is the most common non-viral sexually transmitted infection worldwide, affecting both men and women, though it is often asymptomatic in men.

Trophoblastic Disease

Trophoblastic disease refers to a group of pregnancy-related tumors that arise from the cells that form the placenta, including molar pregnancies and choriocarcinoma. ------ **Interesting FACT**: While most trophoblastic diseases are benign, such as hydatidiform moles, they can become malignant and require chemotherapy.

Tubal Ligation

Tubal ligation, commonly known as "getting your tubes tied," is a surgical procedure in which the fallopian tubes are cut, tied, or sealed to prevent pregnancy.

------ **Interesting FACT**: Tubal ligation is considered a permanent form of birth control, but it can sometimes be reversed, though not always successfully.

Tubal Pregnancy

A tubal pregnancy is a type of ectopic pregnancy in which the fertilized egg implants and grows in a fallopian tube, instead of the uterus, causing life-threatening complications if untreated.

------ **Interesting FACT**: Tubal pregnancies account for over 90% of ectopic pregnancies and often require surgical or medical intervention to prevent rupture and internal bleeding.

Tubo-Ovarian Abscess

A tubo-ovarian abscess is a pus-filled pocket involving the fallopian tube and ovary, often a result of pelvic inflammatory disease (PID) and can lead to infertility if untreated.

------ **Interesting FACT**: Tubo-ovarian abscesses are a medical emergency and typically require antibiotics or surgical drainage to prevent rupture and infection spreading.

Turner Syndrome

Turner syndrome is a genetic disorder that affects females and is caused by the complete or partial absence of one of the X chromosomes, leading to short stature, infertility, and heart defects.

------ **Interesting FACT**: Women with Turner syndrome often undergo hormone replacement therapy to help with growth and the development of secondary sexual characteristics.

Urethral Diverticulum

Urethral diverticulum is a condition where a pouch forms in the urethra, leading to symptoms like pain, urinary tract infections, or discomfort during sexual intercourse.

------ **Interesting FACT**: Urethral diverticulum is often diagnosed through imaging tests like an MRI and may require surgical removal if it causes persistent symptoms.

Urethrovaginal Fistula

A urethrovaginal fistula is an abnormal connection between the urethra and the vagina, often caused by childbirth trauma or surgery, leading to urinary incontinence.

------ **Interesting FACT**: Urethrovaginal fistulas are typically treated with surgical repair, and successful closure restores normal urinary function.

Uterine Abruption

Uterine abruption is a serious complication in which the

placenta detaches from the uterine wall prematurely, depriving the fetus of oxygen and nutrients.

------ **Interesting FACT**: Uterine abruption occurs in about 1% of pregnancies and can lead to heavy bleeding, requiring emergency medical attention to save both the mother and baby.

Uterine Artery Embolization

Uterine artery embolization is a minimally invasive procedure used to treat fibroids by blocking the blood supply to the fibroids, causing them to shrink.

------ **Interesting FACT**: Uterine artery embolization is an alternative to hysterectomy for women who want to avoid surgery and preserve their uterus, though it is not recommended for those who wish to become pregnant.

Uterine Atony

Uterine atony is the failure of the uterus to contract properly after childbirth, leading to postpartum hemorrhage, which is a major cause of maternal mortality.

------ **Interesting FACT**: Uterine atony is typically treated with medications like oxytocin to stimulate contractions or, in severe cases, surgical interventions to control bleeding.

Uterine Cancer

Uterine cancer is a malignant tumor that forms in the tissues of the uterus, most commonly affecting the lining of the uterus (endometrium).

------ **Interesting FACT**: Uterine cancer is the most common gynecological cancer in the United States, with endometrial cancer being the most frequent subtype.

Uterine Fibroids

Uterine fibroids, also known as leiomyomas, are benign tumors that grow in the muscle tissue of the uterus and can cause symptoms like heavy menstrual bleeding, pelvic pain, and pressure.

------ **Interesting FACT**: Fibroids are the most common

type of benign tumor in women and often shrink after menopause due to the decrease in estrogen levels.

Uterine Inversion

Uterine inversion occurs when the uterus turns inside out during or after childbirth, often due to improper management of the third stage of labor, and can lead to severe bleeding.

------ **Interesting FACT**: Uterine inversion is a rare but life-threatening complication, and immediate manual or surgical correction is needed to prevent shock and severe blood loss.

Uterine Polyps

Uterine polyps are growths attached to the inner wall of the uterus that extend into the uterine cavity and can cause irregular menstrual bleeding or infertility.

------ **Interesting FACT**: While uterine polyps are generally benign, they can sometimes turn cancerous, especially in postmenopausal women, which is why they are often removed for analysis.

Uterine Prolapse

Uterine prolapse occurs when the uterus descends into or outside the vaginal canal due to weakened pelvic floor muscles, often causing discomfort and urinary problems.

------ **Interesting FACT**: Uterine prolapse is more common in women who have had multiple vaginal deliveries or who are postmenopausal, and it may require surgical intervention in severe cases.

Uterine Sarcoma

Uterine sarcoma is a rare but aggressive cancer that forms in the muscles or other tissues of the uterus.

------ **Interesting FACT**: Uterine sarcoma accounts for less than 5% of all uterine cancers, but it is more likely to spread quickly compared to other types.

Uterine Septum

A uterine septum is a congenital abnormality where a wall or septum divides the uterus, potentially leading to miscarriages or infertility.

------ **Interesting FACT**: Uterine septum correction through surgery can improve fertility outcomes, particularly for women who have experienced repeated pregnancy losses.

Uterine Sound

A uterine sound is a thin, sterile instrument used to measure the depth of the uterus, often performed during IUD insertion or other gynecological procedures.

------ **Interesting FACT**: Uterine sounding helps ensure that an IUD is placed properly within the uterus and is often a routine part of gynecological exams when intrauterine devices are used.

Uterus Didelphys

Uterus didelphys is a rare congenital condition in which a woman has two uterine cavities, each with its own cervix, and sometimes two vaginas.

------ **Interesting FACT**: Women with uterus didelphys can have normal pregnancies, though there is an increased risk of miscarriage or preterm labor due to the divided uterus.

Vaginal Agenesis

Vaginal agenesis is a rare congenital condition where the vagina is underdeveloped or absent, often associated with conditions like Mayer-Rokitansky-Küster-Hauser syndrome (MRKH).

------ **Interesting FACT**: Women with vaginal agenesis typically have normal ovaries and external genitalia, and surgical procedures can help create a functional vaginal canal.

Vaginal Atrophy

Vaginal atrophy refers to the thinning, drying, and inflammation of the vaginal walls due to a decrease in estrogen, most commonly occurring after menopause.

------ **Interesting FACT**: Vaginal atrophy can cause discomfort during intercourse and frequent urinary tract infections, but hormone replacement therapy and vaginal moisturizers can help manage symptoms.

Vaginal Birth After Cesarean (VBAC)

VBAC refers to a vaginal delivery by a woman who has previously had a cesarean section, an option for many women depending on the type of uterine incision made during the previous cesarean.

------ **Interesting FACT**: VBAC is considered a safe option for many women, with success rates around 60-80%, but not all women are candidates, particularly those with a vertical uterine scar.

Vaginal Cuff

The vaginal cuff is the upper portion of the vagina that is sutured closed after a hysterectomy, where the cervix and uterus are removed.

------ **Interesting FACT**: After a hysterectomy, the vaginal cuff can be a site for complications, such as infections or dehiscence (reopening), but proper post-operative care reduces risks.

Vaginal Vault Prolapse

Vaginal vault prolapse occurs when the top of the vagina loses support and drops after a hysterectomy, sometimes causing discomfort or urinary issues.

------ **Interesting FACT**: Vaginal vault prolapse is often treated surgically, either through sacrocolpopexy or vaginal repair procedures, to restore normal anatomy.

Vaginismus

Vaginismus is the involuntary contraction of the vaginal

muscles, which can make sexual intercourse, pelvic exams, or tampon use painful or impossible.

------ **Interesting FACT**: Vaginismus is often linked to psychological factors such as anxiety or trauma and can be treated with physical therapy, counseling, or gradual desensitization techniques.

Vaginitis

Vaginitis is the inflammation or infection of the vagina, resulting in symptoms like itching, pain, and discharge.

------ **Interesting FACT**: Vaginitis can be caused by various factors, including bacterial infections, yeast infections, or even chemical irritants in soaps and lotions.

Vaginoplasty

Vaginoplasty is a surgical procedure to reconstruct or tighten the vaginal canal, often performed for transgender women or to correct vaginal defects after childbirth or injury.

------ **Interesting FACT**: Vaginoplasty is also used to correct congenital abnormalities, such as vaginal agenesis, and can improve both physical function and appearance.

Vesicovaginal Fistula

A vesicovaginal fistula is an abnormal connection between the bladder and the vagina, often resulting from childbirth trauma or surgery, causing continuous urinary leakage.

------ **Interesting FACT**: Vesicovaginal fistulas are more common in areas with limited access to obstetric care and are usually treated with surgical repair to restore normal function.

Vestibulitis

Vestibulitis is the inflammation of the vestibule, the area surrounding the opening of the vagina, causing pain during intercourse, tampon use, or even sitting.

------ **Interesting FACT**: Vestibulitis is a subtype of vulvodynia, a chronic pain condition affecting the vulvar region, and may require treatment with medications, physical therapy, or surgery.

Vestibulodynia

Vestibulodynia is chronic pain or discomfort localized to the vestibule, the area around the vaginal opening, especially during activities like intercourse or tampon use.
------ **Interesting FACT**: Vestibulodynia is a form of vulvodynia and may be treated with topical medications, physical therapy, or in some cases, surgery.

Vulvar Cancer

Vulvar cancer is a rare type of cancer that affects the external genitalia of women, most commonly the labia. It can present as a lump, sore, or lesion that doesn't heal.
------ **Interesting FACT**: Vulvar cancer is more common in older women and can be caused by human papillomavirus (HPV) infection, particularly strains associated with genital warts.

Vulvar Vestibulitis

Vulvar vestibulitis is an inflammatory condition affecting the vestibule (the area around the vaginal opening), causing pain, burning, or irritation, especially during intercourse or tampon use.

------ **Interesting FACT**: Vulvar vestibulitis is considered a subset of vulvodynia and is thought to be caused by nerve sensitivity or chronic inflammation in the vestibule.

Vulvectomy

A vulvectomy is the surgical removal of all or part of the vulva, often performed to treat vulvar cancer or other conditions affecting the vulva.

------ **Interesting FACT**: Depending on the extent of the surgery, vulvectomy can impact a woman's sexual function and may require reconstructive surgery.

Vulvitis

Vulvitis is the inflammation of the vulva, often caused by

infections, allergies, or irritants such as soaps, and it can lead to itching, redness, and swelling.

------ **Interesting FACT**: Vulvitis is not a specific condition but a symptom of various underlying issues, including yeast infections or contact dermatitis from hygiene products.

Vulvodynia

Vulvodynia is chronic pain or discomfort around the vulva with no identifiable cause, often affecting sexual activity and quality of life.

------ **Interesting FACT**: Vulvodynia affects up to 16% of women, yet its causes remain largely unknown, making it challenging to treat.

Vulvovaginitis

Vulvovaginitis is the inflammation of the vulva and vagina, often caused by infections, allergens, or irritants, leading to itching, pain, and abnormal discharge.

------ **Interesting FACT**: Vulvovaginitis can result from a variety of causes, including yeast infections, bacterial vaginosis, or contact dermatitis from products like soaps or detergents.

Wilms' Tumor

Wilms' tumor is a rare kidney cancer that primarily affects children, but in gynecology, it can sometimes be confused with masses or tumors in the pelvic region during diagnosis.

------ **Interesting FACT**: Wilms' tumor is highly treatable, with a survival rate of over 90% when detected early, and treatment usually involves surgery and chemotherapy.

Zona Pellucida

The zona pellucida is a thick, transparent outer layer surrounding an ovum (egg), which must be penetrated by sperm during fertilization.

------ **Interesting FACT**: The zona pellucida plays a critical role in preventing polyspermy, the fertilization of an egg by more than one sperm, by undergoing changes once the egg is fertilized.

Zygosity

Zygosity refers to the genetic similarity between twins, where monozygotic (identical) twins come from the same fertilized egg, while dizygotic (fraternal) twins come from two separate eggs.

------ **Interesting FACT**: Monozygotic twins share the same DNA, while dizygotic twins are no more genetically similar than regular siblings, although they share the same womb.

Zygote Intrafallopian Transfer (ZIFT)

ZIFT is an assisted reproductive technology (ART) procedure in which a fertilized egg (zygote) is placed into a woman's fallopian tube instead of the uterus, as in standard IVF.

------ **Interesting FACT**: ZIFT is less commonly used than traditional IVF, as it requires laparoscopic surgery to transfer the zygote to the fallopian tube.

Zygote

A zygote is the single cell formed when a sperm fertilizes an egg, marking the earliest stage of human development.

------ **Interesting FACT**: After fertilization, the zygote undergoes rapid cell division, becoming a blastocyst that implants into the uterine wall to begin pregnancy.

About the Author

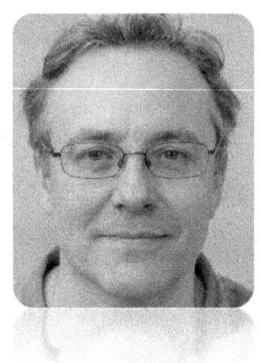

Damian O. Cook is a dedicated author specializing in books that simplify complex medical terms across various fields. With a clear and accessible writing style, Damian's work makes understanding medical terminology easy for readers of all backgrounds, from students to healthcare professionals. His books offer straightforward explanations and interesting insights, making essential knowledge available to everyone.